Low Carb Cookbook For Beginners and Pros

Your Essential Guide to Living the Low Carb Lifestyle - Healthy and Delicious Recipes for Every Day incl. 14 Days Meal Plan

Marc C. Goodwin

ISBN - 9798795714981

Table of Contents

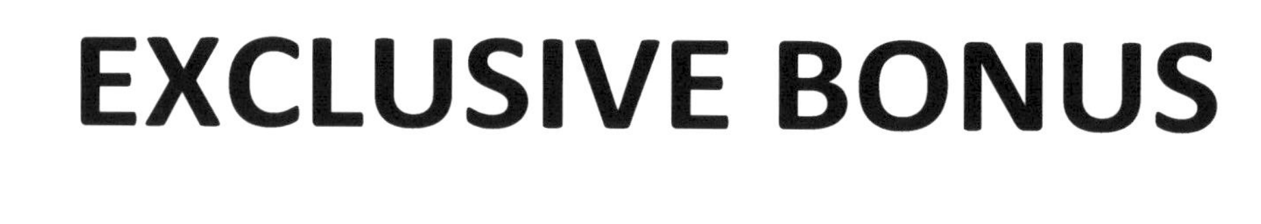

40 Weight Loss Recipes

&

14 Days Meal Plan

Scan the QR-Code and receive
the FREE download:

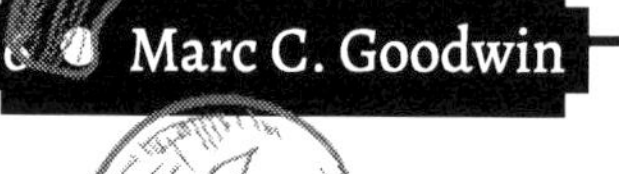

Introduction to Low-Carbohydrate Diets

What is a Low-Carbohydrate Diet?

Low-carbohydrate diets (also known as low-carb diets or carb-restricted diets) are pretty self-explanatory. They refer to diets that contain very few carbohydrates compared to an average diet.

There are three main macronutrients - carbohydrates, proteins, and fats. In a low-carb diet, high-carb foods are avoided. This includes foods like wheat, bran, oats, potatoes, and ultra-processed foods.

Because you are cutting out all of these major foods when you follow the low-carb diet, you naturally begin to eat more proteins and fats. The high-carb foods that were once in your diet get replaced with either lower carbohydrate foods, or protein-rich and fat-rich foods, such as meats, fish, dairy, fruits, vegetables, nuts, and seeds.

It's important to note that the aim with low-carb diets is not to completely cut out the macronutrient. You will still be eating some carbohydrates. As a general rule of thumb, low-crab diets require you to eat fewer than 130 grams of carbohydrates each day. The carbohydrates that you consume will come from healthy sources. This ensures that you are still eating adequate amounts of fibre, vitamins, and minerals.

Who Are Low-Carb Diets Suitable For?

Low-carb diets aren't for everyone. In fact, they might be inappropriate for some people, depending on your individual needs and circumstances. Before you decide to start a low-carb diet or make any drastic changes to your diet, you should consult your doctor or dietitian beforehand. They will give you their expert advice and may be able to guide you through the process.

However, the low-carb diet can be extremely beneficial for many people. We will cover more of the benefits of the low-carb diet later on in this book, but low-carb diets are particularly beneficial for the following groups of people:

- People who suffer from type 1 diabetes
- People who are looking to lose weight
- People who have an upcoming long-distance athletic event
- People with high blood pressure or high blood cholesterol levels

If you're thinking about starting on a low-carb diet and you're looking for some guidance, this recipe book is perfect for you! We're going to cover everything you need to know about going low-carb, including the types of low-carb diets, what foods you can and can't eat, and common mistakes to avoid when you're low-carb.

After we've covered the basics of low-carb diets, we're going to give you a range of different low-carb recipes that you can create for breakfast, lunch, dinner, and snacks. Every recipe is made with simple ingredients that you can find in any UK, US, or Canadian store, and they're great for beginners or pros in the kitchen. We've also added the nutritional values (including the calories, and the carb, protein, and fat content) for every recipe so that you can track your intake accurately.

At the end of the book, we'll give you a 14 days meal plan. This is the perfect plan for you to follow during the first two weeks of your low-carb journey. You can use the meal plan as a guide until you feel comfortable trying out your own nutrition plan! The meal-plan contains additional recipes to those that are listed in this book so you've got lots of variety in your low-carb diet!

What Are the Benefits of Low-Carb Diets?

Eating a low amount of carbohydrates in your diet can provide a range of health benefits, including the ones below.

They Decrease Your Appetite

If you're trying to lose weight or cut out the processed food, the hunger can be difficult to deal with. In fact, it's one of the most common reasons why people give up on their diets after just a couple of weeks.

Low-carb diets may help to combat your hunger pangs. When you're eating more protein and fat, you will naturally feel fuller after your meals.

They Can Enhance Weight Loss

Cutting carbohydrates out of your diet is one of the best ways to lose weight. Simply removing the starchy foods from your diet can cut your calories and make it easier to achieve a calorie deficit.

Studies show that those who eat a low-carb diet lose more weight and lose it quicker than those who eat a high-carb, low-fat diet. The reason for this is because carbohydrates tend to hold onto water in your body. When you reduce your carb intake, your water carries less water.

This results in weight loss. It's important to note that the differences in weight loss between low-carb and low-fat diets is similar after a few months of dieting.

They Can Lower Blood Pressure

High blood pressure, known medically as hypertension, is a significant risk factor for a range of different health conditions, including heart disease, stroke, type 2 diabetes, and kidney disease.

Eating a low-carb diet can reduce your blood pressure and, therefore, reduce your risk of developing these diseases.

They Improve Your Blood Cholesterol Levels

When you consume simple sugars, it can cause your blood triglyceride levels to increase a lot. Low-carb diets help to decrease the levels of triglycerides in your blood, which can also decrease your risk of developing heart disease.

Additionally, eating fewer carbohydrates each day can help to decrease the levels of low-density lipoproteins (LDLs) in your blood. LDLs are known as the 'bad' cholesterol because they can increase plaque build-up in your arteries, which increases your risk of atherosclerosis and heart disease.

Low-carb diets can also increase the levels of high-density lipoproteins (HDLs) in your blood. HDLs are the 'good' cholesterol that have the opposite effect to LDLs and lower the risk of plaque build up.

They Can Help to Regulate Your Blood Sugar Levels

If you suffer from type 1 or type 2 diabetes, eating a low-carb diet can be extremely helpful. Medical professionals and nutritionists often prescribe low-carb diets to those with a diabetes diagnosis because it can help to decrease blood insulin levels.

This is because when you eat carbohydrates, it causes your blood glucose (blood sugar) levels to increase. This stimulates the production of insulin in the pancreas and causes a huge insulin spike in the blood, which can be dangerous in those with type 2 diabetes.

Low-carb diets can reduce required insulin dosage by 50% in those with type 1 diabetes, too.

They Can Benefit Your Brain

Believe it or now, low-carb diets can even boost your brain health! Your brain's primary source of energy is glucose, and some parts of your brain can't use any other energy form apart from glucose.

When you're not eating enough glucose (carbohydrates) in your diet, your liver will form glucose from amino acids and fatty acids so that these parts of your brain can continue to function optimally.

The parts of your brain that can use alternative energy sources will burn ketones for fuel when glucose levels are low. When your body is burning ketones for energy, this is known as being in a state of ketosis.

Studies show that being in ketosis can boost brain function and may decrease the risk of neurodegenerative diseases, such as Alzheimer's disease and Parkinson's disease. Ketosis has also been beneficial in reducing seizure rates in children with epilepsy.

What Foods Should You Eat in Low-Carb Diets?

To help you achieve a low number of carbohydrates each day, there are certain foods that you should focus. In particular, look out for foods that are high in proteins and healthy fats.

Here is a quick list of some great low-carb foods that you can include in your diet:

- Meats – chicken, turkey, grass-fed beef, pork, lamb, and duck
- Fish – salmon, cod, haddock, white fish, and tuna
- Dairy – eggs, cheese, yoghurt, and milk
- Non-dairy alternatives – tofu, tempeh, dairy-free cheese, dairy-free yoghurts, and various nut milks
- Fruits – apples, oranges, strawberries, blueberries, pears, peaches

- Vegetables – almost every vegetable is appropriate, apart from starchy vegetables (see below). Aim to include lots of broccoli, cauliflower, carrots, sprouts, spinach, and kale in your diet
- Nuts and seeds – almonds, cashews, walnuts, pistachios, brazil nuts, hazelnuts, sunflower seeds, pumpkin seeds, chia seeds
- Oils – olive oil, coconut oil, fish oil, grass-fed butter
- Drinks – water, sparkling water, coffee, and tea. Be careful not to add a lot of sugar to your hot drinks, as this will increase your carb intake

Although these foods are welcomed in low-carb diets, it's important to remember that some of these foods contain a lot of calories. If you're trying to lose weight, be careful not to overconsume dairy, nuts, seeds, and oils. Doing so can significantly increase your calories and might make it harder for you to lose weight.

You can eat the following foods in moderate amounts.

- Starchy vegetables – white potatoes, sweet potatoes, parsnips, turnips, and swede
- Grains – brown rice, wholemeal pasta, oats, quinoa, and buckwheat
- Legumes – lentils, kidney beans, white beans, black beans, and pinto beans
- Dark chocolate – choose brands that contain at least 75% cocoa

You'll need to be careful not to exceed your carbohydrate limit (130 grams) if you include these foods in your diet because they all contain moderate-high amounts of carbohydrates.

What Foods Should Be Avoided in Low-Carb Diets?

Now we've gone through everything that you can eat on a low-carb diet, let's go through what you should try and avoid on this type of diet.

Basically, any food that is very high in carbohydrates is better avoided in any type of low-carb diet. The reasons for this are fairly obvious, but if you have a limit of 130 grams of carbohydrates a day, you don't want to 'waste' all of those on just one piece of food.

For example, an average medium-sized white potato contains around 90 grams of carbohydrates. Therefore, if you ate a medium white potato on a low-carb diet, you'd only have 40 grams of carbohydrates left to consume for the rest of the day. To put it into perspective, that equates to just two slices of bread!

You're much better avoiding the foods that contain a lot of carbohydrates so that you can spread the limited amount of carbohydrates that you can have throughout the whole day. This will give you more sustained energy and will help you to feel fuller and more satiated.

So, what foods should you stay away from when you're on a low-carb diet? Here are some of the key foods to avoid.

- Refined grains – wheat, barley, rye, pasta, bread, cereal
- Sugar – processed snacks (sweetened chocolate, candy, ice cream, cookies), pastries, honey, agave, and sweetened soft drinks or sodas
- Trans fats – hydrogenated or partially hydrogenated oils

- Starchy vegetables – white potatoes, sweet potatoes, and parsnips
- Low-fat products – such as low-fat spreads or snacks. Food manufacturers often replace the fat with sugars or sweeteners

Common Mistakes in Low-Carb Diets

Here are some of the common mistakes that many people make when they are trying to follow a low-carb diet.

Eating Too Many Carbohydrates

By far, the most common mistake that people make when following any sort of low-carb diet is eating too many carbs.

It's surprisingly easier to over-consume this macronutrient because there are hidden carbs in so many different foods that we know and love. Before we've even realised it, we've eaten way more than 130 grams of carbs and we're exceeded our carb limit!

Most traditional Western diets contain a lot more carbs than 130 grams. So, when you initially start your low-crab diet, it can be difficult to stick to the limit, especially if you're usually a carb lover!

As long as you stick to the foods mentioned above and avoid the high-carb items, you should find it fairly easy to stick to 130 grams of carbs a day or less.

Being Inpatient

Being in a low-carb diet can provide a range of benefits. But it takes time to see positive changes in your physical and mental health. You need to be patient if you want to make significant progress.

For example, if your goal is weight loss, it will take at least a few months to start seeing significant changes on the scale. Stick to your low-carb diet and be patient, and you will see the results that you're after!

Giving Up

If you're used to eating a diet that is high in carbohydrates, it might be pretty difficult to stick to your new low-carb diet. It takes a week or two for your body to acclimatise to your new food intake.

During this time, your body is switching from using carbs as a primary fuel source to using fats and proteins instead. This can be a difficult time, and this is where many people give up!

Eating Too Much Protein

Even though you will naturally eat more protein when you're on a low-carb diet, you can end up eating too much.

The issue is that protein is the most satiating macronutrient, meaning it keeps you full for the longest. This is great if your goal is to lose weight, but if you eat large volumes of protein, you can end up feeling overly full and bloated.

Excess proteins get converted into glucose via a process called gluconeogenesis. This is not ideal if you're on a low-carb diet because you want to keep your glucose levels to a minimum.

Eating Too Few Carbohydrates

When you're trying to go low carb, it's quite easy to over the top. You can end up eating too few carbs each day.

There's a huge difference between 'low-carb' and 'no carb'. You want to aim for around 100-150 grams of carbs every day. No more and no less! It's just as detrimental under consuming your carbs than it is over consuming them.

Being Worried About Eating Too Much Fat

Eating a higher fat diet can be intimidating, especially when media focuses so much on everything being low-fat. Many people get around about eating these extra fats, but it's what the body needs to replace the carbohydrates you're lacking.

Focus on eating lots of healthy fat sources to ensure you get plenty of omega-3s and omega-6s. Your fats should account for 60-70% of your total calorie intake.

Low-Carb Recipes

Low-Carb Breakfasts

Low-Carb Breakfast Waffles

Makes 4 servings
Preparation time - 5 minutes
Cooking time - 5 minutes
Nutritional values per serving - 359 kcals, 15 g carbs, 19 g protein, 17 g fat

Ingredients

For the waffles:

- 6 eggs
- 2 bananas, mashed
- 2 tbsp peanut butter or almond butter
- 3 tbsp wholemeal flour
- 1/2 tsp ground cinnamon

For the toppings:

- 1/2 tbsp cashew butter
- 1/2 tbsp coconut butter
- 4 medium strawberries
- 1 tsp honey or maple syrup

Method

1. Heat a waffle iron until hot.
2. Meanwhile, mix all of the waffle ingredients in a large bowl until they form a smooth and consistent mixture
3. Coat the waffle iron with cooking spray and pour 1/4 of the batter into the iron.
4. Cook for a few minutes until golden.
5. Repeat this a further three times to create four delicious waffles.
6. Serve warm with the cashew butter, coconut butter, strawberries, and honey on top.

Bacon and Egg Rolls

Makes 4 servings
Preparation time - 10 minutes
Cooking time - 10 minutes
Nutritional values per serving - 313 kcals, 9 g carbs, 17 g protein, 25 g fat

Ingredients

- 6 eggs, beaten
- 2 tbsp milk (any type)
- 1/2 tsp garlic powder
- 1/4 tsp black pepper
- 1 tbsp salted butter
- 12 slices bacon
- 80 g / 3 oz cheddar cheese, grated

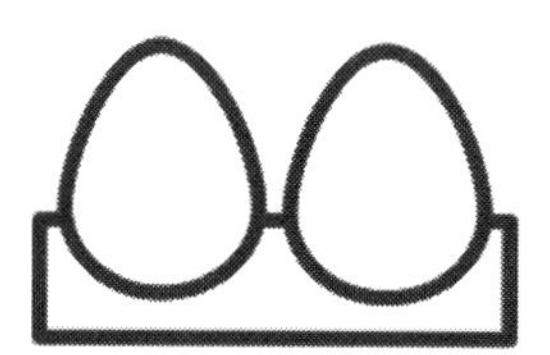

Method

1. In a large bowl, whisk the eggs, milk, garlic powder, and pepper until combined.
2. Heat the butter in a skillet. When melted, add the egg mixture, and cook for 3-4 minutes, stirring regularly to form a scramble.
3. Place the bacon slices flat on a chopping board and spread half of the cheddar cheese evenly across the bottom third of each slice. Top the cheese with half of the egg scramble.
4. Repeat with the remaining halves of cheese and egg scramble until all of the ingredients have been used.
5. Carefully roll up the bacon slices, keeping the cheese and egg mixture tightly inside.
6. Add the bacon rolls to the hot skillet and cook for 5 minutes of either side until the bacon turns dark and crispy.
7. Serve immediately.

Keto Bagels

Makes 8 servings
Preparation time - 15 minutes
Cooking time - 20 minutes
Nutritional values per serving - 245 kcals, 15 g carbs, 10 g protein, 29 g fat

Ingredients

- 250 g / 9 oz almond flour
- 1 tbsp baking powder
- 250 g / 9 oz mozzarella cheese, grated
- 100 g / 3.5 oz cream cheese
- 2 eggs, beaten
- 1/2 tsp chia seeds
- 1/2 tsp black pepper
- 1 tbsp butter

Method

1. Preheat the oven to 200 °C / 400 °F and line a baking tray with parchment paper.
2. Meanwhile, combine the almond flour and baking powder in a bowl.
3. Add the mozzarella to a heat proof bowl and gradually heat in the microwave for 30 seconds at a time until fully melted. This should take around 1 ½ to 2 minutes.
4. Stir the cream cheese into the melted mozzarella and heat in the microwave for a further 30 seconds.
5. Scrape the melted cheese mixture into the flour and baking powder mixture. Stir in the beaten eggs until it forms a dough-like mixture.
6. Split the dough into 8 equal balls and press your finger into the centre of each ball to form bagel shapes.
7. Place the bagels on the baking sheet and sprinkle with chia seeds and black pepper. You might need to press the seeds and pepper into the dough so that they don't fall off while the bagels are baking.
8. Bake in the oven for 20 minutes until the dough is cooked all the way through and golden on top.

Vegetable Frittata

Makes 8 servings
Preparation time - 15 minutes
Cooking time - 60 minutes
Nutritional values per serving - 415 kcals, 11 g carbs, 19 g protein, 22 g fat

Ingredients

- 8 slices bacon
- 1/2 onion, finely sliced
- 100 g / 3.5 oz spinach, chopped
- 1/2 red bell pepper, sliced
- 12 large eggs, beaten
- 200 ml milk (cow's milk or cashew milk)
- 1/2 tsp salt
- 100 g / 3.5 oz cheddar cheese, grated

Method

1. Preheat the oven to 200 °C / 400 °F and line a baking tray with parchment paper and grease a cake tin with butter or oil.
2. Heat a sauté pan on a high temperature and add the bacon slices. Cook for 10 minutes until crispy and browned. Once cooked, remove from the pan and place on kitchen roll to drain.
3. Add the onions and pepper to the pan and cook for 5 minutes until soft.
4. In a bowl, whisk together the eggs, milk, and salt until combined.
5. Chop the bacon into small pieces and stir into the egg mixture along with the onions and peppers.
6. Pour the mixture into the greased cake tin and sprinkle the cheddar cheese evenly across the top.
7. Bake in the oven for 20 minutes until the frittata is fully cooked and the cheese is melted and golden.
8. Allow to cool for 10-15 minutes before cutting into slices.

Strawberry and Avocado Low-Fat Smoothie

Makes 1 serving
Preparation time - 5 minutes
Cooking time - none
Nutritional values per serving - 106 kcals, 6 g carbs, 10 g protein, 12 g fat

Ingredients

- 200 g / 7 oz strawberries
- 1 avocado
- 200 ml non-dairy milk (almond, cashew, hazelnut, soya, or oat)

Method

1. Remove the greens from the strawberries and chop them in half.
2. Peel the avocado and remove the pit. Chopped into small chunks.
3. Add all of the ingredients to a blender or food processor.
4. Pulse until the ingredients are fully combined.
5. Serve in your favourite glass and enjoy!

Cashew Butter Breakfast Pots

Makes 1 serving
Preparation time - 10 minutes
Cooking time - none
Nutritional values per serving - 236 kcals, 26 g carbs, 19 g protein, 13 g fat

Ingredients

- 5 strawberries, halved
- 2 tbsp peanut butter
- 1 tbsp jam
- 3 tbsp Greek yoghurt
- 30 g / 1 oz granola
- 30 g / 1 oz chopped mixed nuts (almonds, cashews, walnuts, or hazelnuts)
- 1 tsp chia seeds

Method

1. In a tall glass, place half of the strawberries and top with 1 tbsp peanut butter.
2. Add 1 tbsp jam, 1 tbsp Greek yoghurt, and half of the granola in layers on top of the strawberries and peanut butter.
3. Repeat steps 1 and 2.
4. After the final layer of granola has been added to the glass, finish with the final scoop of Greek yoghurt, the chopped nuts, and the chia seeds
5. Serve immediately while the yoghurt is still fresh.

Egg and Vegetable Bowl

Makes 2 servings
Preparation time - 5 minutes
Cooking time - 20 minutes
Nutritional values per serving - 213 kcals, 11 g carbs, 18 g protein, 14 g fat

Ingredients

- 100 g / 3.5 oz baby new potato, halved
- 1 tbsp olive oil
- 1 courgette, diced
- 1 red pepper, sliced
- 1 onion, finely sliced
- 1 garlic clove, peeled and crushed
- 1 tbsp dried mixed herbs
- 4 eggs

Method

1. Bring a saucepan of water to boil and add the potatoes. Cook for 10 minutes until soft.
2. Heat the olive oil in a large frying pan and add the courgette, pepper, onion, and garlic. Cook for 10 minutes until the vegetables begin to soften and turn brown.
3. Make 4 holes in the pan and crack an egg into each. Continue cooking until egg whites have cooked and the yolks are still soft.
4. Serve with a side of low-carb bread or a side salad.

Low-Carb Lunches

Chicken and Veggie Bowls

Makes 4 servings
Preparation time - 45 minutes
Cooking time - 30 minutes
Nutritional values per serving - 231 kcals, 6 g carbs, 23 g protein, 9 g fat

Ingredients

- 400 g / 14 oz chicken breast fillets, diced
- 2 tbsp soy sauce
- 1 tbsp olive oil
- 100 g / 3.5 oz broccoli, chopped into small pieces
- 100 g / 3.5 oz carrots, thinly sliced
- 4 tbsp sweet corn

Method

1. Place the diced chicken breast pieces into a large mixing bowl and add the soy sauce. Toss to coat the chicken and cover with tin foil. Set aside for 30 minutes to marinade.
2. Heat the olive oil in a frying pan and add the chicken. Cook for 15 minutes until it is cooked and golden. Add broccoli and carrots and cook for a further 5 minutes until the vegetables have softened.
3. Remove from the heat and evenly serve the chicken and vegetables into four bowls.
4. Stir 1 tbsp of the sweetcorn into each bowl and enjoy.

Deliciously Devilled Eggs

Makes 4 servings
Preparation time - 20 minutes
Cooking time - 15 minutes
Nutritional values per serving - 212 kcals, 7 g carbs, 16 g protein, 30 g fat

Ingredients

- 8 large eggs, whole
- 3 tbsp mayonnaise
- 1 tsp Dijon mustard
- 1 tsp apple cider vinegar
- 1/2 tsp salt
- 1/2 tsp black pepper

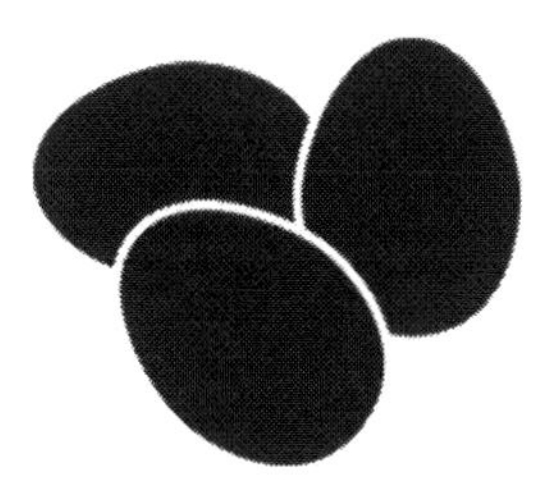

Method

1. Fill a saucepan with water and bring to boil. Reduce the heat to low and carefully place the eggs in the water.
2. Bring the heat back up to a boil and leave to cook for 12-15 minutes.
3. Once cooked, turn the heat off, remove the eggs from the pan, and set aside to cool.
4. When the eggs are cool enough, peel the shells off and remove the yolks using a spoon. Try to keep the egg whites whole while you do this. Set the egg whites to the side.
5. In a bowl, mix the yolks together with the mayonnaise, mustard, apple cider vinegar, salt, and pepper until fully combined.
6. Place the eggs whites on a serving plate or tray and spoon the yolk mixture into the whole of each one.
7. Add an extra sprinkle of black pepper to taste.

Steak Bites and Zucchini Noodles

Makes 4 servings
Preparation time - 15 minutes
Cooking time - 15 minutes
Nutritional values per serving - 331 kcals, 9 g carbs, 20 g protein, 8 g fat

Ingredients

- 3 tbsp olive oil
- 4 garlic cloves, peeled and minced
- 1 tbsp soy sauce
- 1/2 tsp garlic powder
- 1/2 tsp paprika
- 1/2 tsp black pepper
- 500 g / 18 oz sirloin steak, diced
- 3 zucchinis, spiralized

Method

1. In a frying pan, heat 2 tbsp olive oil and add the garlic. Cook for 5 minutes until fragrant.
2. Stir in the soy sauce garlic powder, paprika, and black pepper. Set aside to cool while you prepare the rest of the dish.
3. Heat the remaining 1 tbsp olive oil in the pan and add the diced steak. Cook for 3/4 minutes on each side until the steak is almost cooked.
4. Pour the sauce into the pan and continue cooking for 1 further minute, stirring to fully coat the steak in the sauce.
5. Heat the zucchini noodles if desired or serve them cold alongside the steak bites.

Avocado, Egg, and Tomato Salad

Makes 4 servings
Preparation time - 10 minutes
Cooking time - 20 minutes
Nutritional values per serving - 112 kcals, 8 g carbs, 6 g protein, 12 g fat

Ingredients

- 8 eggs
- 1 tbsp olive oil
- 8 strips bacon
- 2 tbsp mayonnaise
- 5 tbsp Greek yoghurt
- 1/2 tsp black pepper
- 1 avocado
- 50 g / 1.8 oz feta cheese, grated
- 8 cherry tomatoes, halved
- Handful lettuce

Method

1. Heat a saucepan of water and bring to boil. Add the eggs and cook for 10 minutes until hard-boiled. Set aside to cool before peeling and halving.
2. Heat 1 tbsp olive oil in a skillet and add the bacon strips. Cook for 8-10 minutes, turning hallway through, until brown and crispy.
3. Set the bacon aside to drain on paper towels.
4. In a bowl, combine the mayonnaise, Greek yoghurt, and black pepper.
5. Peel the avocado and slice thinly. Add to the bowl and stir to coat in the sauce.
6. Place a bed of lettuce on the bottom of each bowl and add half an egg to each, following by 2 slices of bacon, cherry tomatoes, and a sprinkle of grated feta cheese.
7. Add a dollop of sauce onto each salad and toss to coat the other ingredients.
8. Enjoy the salad for lunch.

Chicken with Parmesan and Mushrooms

Makes 4 servings
Preparation time - 10 minutes
Cooking time - 30 minutes
Nutritional values per serving - 318 kcals, 8 g carbs, 14 g protein, 16 g fat

Ingredients

- 2 tbsp olive oil
- 400 g / 14 oz skinless, boneless chicken thighs
- 1 tsp salt
- 1 tsp black pepper
- 200 g / 7 oz mushroom, sliced
- 4 garlic cloves, peeled and minced
- 200 ml whipping cream
- 100 g / 3.5 oz Parmesan cheese
- 1 tsp dried mixed herbs

Method

1. Heat 2 tbsp olive oil in a large skillet and add the chicken thighs, salt, and black pepper. Cook for 10-12 minutes until golden and crispy.
2. Remove the chicken and place on paper towels to drain. Leave the chicken juices in the pan.
3. Add the mushrooms and garlic to the pan and cook for 5 minutes until softened.
4. Reduce the heat and add the whipping cream. Simmer for 10 minutes, stirring frequently.
5. Add the Parmesan cheese to the skillet and heat until melted.
6. Return the chicken to the skillet and stir to coat in the cheese mixture.
7. Serve hot with a side of vegetables.

Bacon Sushi Rolls

Makes 8 servings
Preparation time - 10 minutes
Cooking time - 20 minutes
Nutritional values per serving - 112 kcals, 6 g carbs, 8 g protein, 15 g fat

Ingredients

- 1 tbsp olive oil
- 4 slices bacon
- 1 cucumber
- 2 carrots,
- 1 avocado
- 100 g / 3.5 oz cream cheese

Method

1. Heat the olive oil in a skillet and cook the bacon for 4-5 minutes until crispy and brown. Set aside to drain on paper towels.
2. Cut the cucumber, carrots, and avocado into thin strips that are the same width and thickness as the bacon slices.
3. Spread a layer of cream cheese along each strip of bacon and layer with cucumber, carrot, and avocado slices. Repeat until all of the vegetables are used.
4. Roll each slice of bacon up tightly into a sushi roll and serve warm or cold.

Stuffed Avocados

Makes 2 servings
Preparation time - 10 minutes
Cooking time - 5 minutes
Nutritional values per serving - 112 kcals, 8 g carbs, 6 g protein, 12 g fat

Ingredients

- 2 medium avocados
- 2 slices bacon
- 4 cherry tomatoes, halved
- 1 tsp lemon or lime juice
- 1/2 tsp garlic powder
- 1/2 tsp black pepper

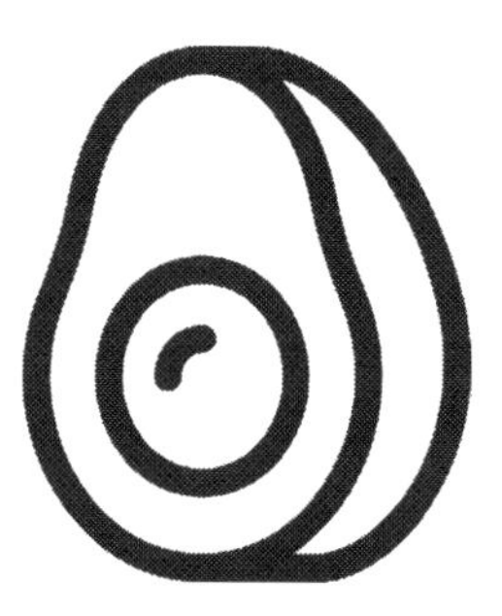

Method

1. Heat a skillet and add the bacon slices. Cook for 5 minutes on either side until the edges begin to curl and the bacon begins to brown and turn crispy.
2. Once cooked, set the bacon aside to drain on some paper towels.
3. Peel the avocadoes, and slice down the middle so that each one forms two even halves. Remove the pits, trying to keep each avocado untouched.
4. Slice the cooked bacon into small pieces and place in a bowl. Add the halved cherry tomatoes, 1 tsp lemon or lime juice, and garlic powder. Mix to combine.
5. Spoon the mixture into the holes of each avocado half and sprinkle some black pepper over the top of each.

Chicken and Vegetables with Tzatziki

Makes 4 servings
Preparation time - 1 hour 20 minutes
Cooking time - 30 minutes
Nutritional values per serving - 345 kcals, 10 g carbs, 18 g protein, 15 g fat

Ingredients

For the tzatziki:

- 2 cucumbers, peeled and shredded
- 100 ml full-fat Greek yoghurt
- 4 tbsp mayonnaise
- 2 garlic cloves, minced

For the marinade:

- 2 tbsp olive oil
- Juice 1 lemon
- 2 garlic cloves, minced
- 1 tbsp dried mixed herbs
- 1 tsp paprika
- 1 tsp salt
- 1 tsp black pepper

For the chicken and vegetables:

- 400 g / 14 oz skinless, boneless chicken breast
- 2 large aubergines, cubed
- 8 cherry tomatoes, halved

Method

1. To make the tzatziki, mix all of the ingredients in a bowl until combined. Set aside
2. For the marinade, mix all of the ingredients together. Add the chicken, aubergine, and tomatoes to the bowl, and toss to fully coat.
3. Leave the chicken and vegetables to marinade for 1 hour.
4. Preheat the oven to 200 °C / 400 °F and line a baking tray with parchment paper and grease a cake tin with butter or oil.
5. Place the chicken and vegetables evenly on the lined baking tray and cook for 30 minutes until the chicken is golden and crispy.
6. Remove from the oven and serve with the tzatziki.

Tuscan Salmon

Makes 4 servings
Preparation time - 10 minutes
Cooking time - 20 minutes
Nutritional values per serving - 341 kcals, 12 g carbs, 16 g protein, 19 g fat

Ingredients

- 2 tbsp olive oil
- 400 g / 14 oz salmon fillets
- 4 garlic cloves, peeled and minced
- 1 onion, sliced
- 1 vegetable stock cube
- 100 g / 3.5 oz sun-dried tomatoes, drained
- 100 ml heavy cream
- ½ tsp salt
- ½ tsp black pepper
- 200 g / 7 oz spinach
- 100 g / 3.5 oz Parmesan cheese, grated

Method

1. Heat 1 tbsp olive oil in a large frying pan and cook the salmon fillets for 10 minutes, turning halfway through. Once cooked, set aside to drain on paper towels.
2. In the same pan, heat the second tbsp of olive oil and add the garlic and onion. Fry for 5-7 minutes until soft and fragrant.
3. Dissolve the vegetable stock cube according to the packet instructions and add to the frying pan.
4. Reduce the heat to a gentle simmer and stir in the heavy cream. Add the salt and black pepper to season.
5. Add the spinach to the pan and continue heating for 3-4 minutes until the spinach begins to wilt.
6. Stir in the grated Parmesan cheese and continue stirring until melted.
7. Serve the salmon with the hot cheese sauce over the top. Add a side of steamed vegetables and enjoy.

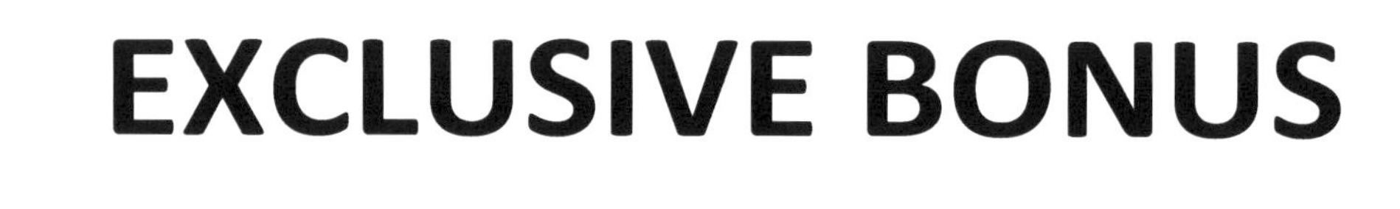

EXCLUSIVE BONUS

40 Weight Loss Recipes

&

14 Days Meal Plan

Scan the QR-Code and receive
the FREE download:

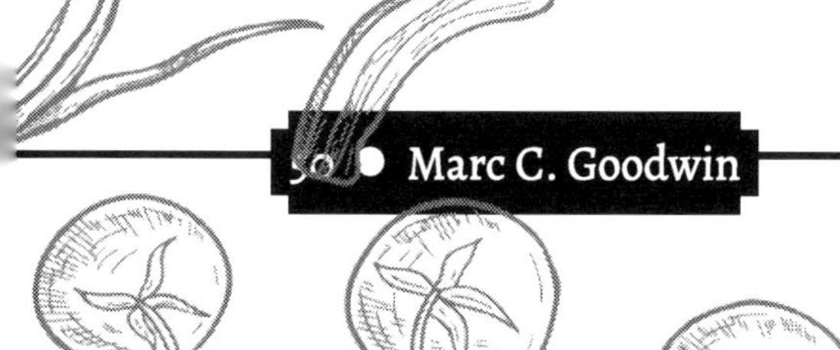

Low-Carb Dinners

Steak and Cheese Stuffed Peppers

Makes 2 servings
Preparation time - 10 minutes
Cooking time - 50 minutes
Nutritional values per serving - 278 kcals, 19 g carbs, 18 g protein, 25 g fat

Ingredients

- 4 large red bell peppers, halved and deseeded
- 1 tbsp olive oil
- 1 onion, sliced
- 200 g / 7 oz button mushrooms, halved
- 200 g / 7 oz steak strips, thinly sliced
- 1 tbsp dried herbs
- 1/2 tsp salt
- 1/2 tsp black pepper
- 1 tbsp soy sauce
- 100 g / 3.5 oz cheddar cheese, grated

Method

1. Preheat the oven to 200 °C / 400 °F and line a baking tray with parchment paper and grease a cake tin with butter or oil.
2. Place the peppers on the baking tray and bake for 20-30 minutes until the edges are beginning to turn brown and crispy.
3. Meanwhile, heat the olive oil in a large skillet over medium heat. Add the onion and cook for 5 minutes until they start to soften and turn brown. Add the mushrooms and cook for a further 5 minutes until they start to release water.
4. Add the steak, herbs, salt, and black pepper to the pan and cook for 4-5 minutes, stirring constantly.
5. Pour the soy sauce into the pan and stir for 30-60 seconds to coat the ingredients.
6. Pour the steak mixture evenly into each pepper and top with the cheddar cheese.
7. Bake in the oven for 10 minutes until the cheese has melted.
8. Serve for dinner while still warm with a side of low-carb vegetables.

Low-Carb Sausage Pizza

Makes 4 servings
Preparation time - 10 minutes
Cooking time - 15 minutes
Nutritional values per serving - 510 kcals, 15 g carbs, 20 g protein, 25 g fat

Ingredients

For the crust:

- 100 g / 3.5 oz mozzarella cheese, grated
- 2 tbsp cream cheese
- 200 g / 7 oz almond flour
- 1 egg, beaten
- 1 tsp salt

For the toppings:

- 1 tsp olive oil
- 1 sausage, sliced
- 2 tbsp tomato paste
- 1 tsp dried mixed herbs
- 50 g / 1.8 oz mozzarella cheese, grated

Method

1. Preheat the oven to 200 °C / 400 °F and line a pizza tray with parchment paper or use butter to grease it.
2. Heat the mozzarella and cream cheese in a saucepan in a pan over medium heat, stirring frequently.
3. Stir in the almond flour, egg, and salt until combined.
4. Flatten the dough on a clean surface and transfer to the lined pizza tray to around an 8-inch diameter circle.
5. Bake in the oven for 10 minutes until the crust has hardened slightly and has turned golden brown.
6. While the dough is cooking, heat 1 tbsp oil in a frying pan and sauté the sausage for 5-7 minutes until they are fully cooked on both sides.
7. Spread the tomato paste across the pizza and top with the cheese, sausage, and herbs.
8. Bake in the oven for a further 10 minutes until the cheese has melted.
9. Serve with a side salad or some low-carb vegetables.

Spicy Fish Taco Bowls

Makes 4 servings
Preparation time - 15 minutes
Cooking time - 15 minutes
Nutritional values per serving - 467 kcals, 22 g carbs, 30 g protein, 5 g fat

Ingredients

- 1 tsp chilli powder
- 1 tsp smoked paprika
- 1/2 tsp cayenne pepper
- 1/2 tsp salt
- 1 tbsp olive oil
- 2 cloves garlic, minced
- 4 white fish fillets
- 1 onion, sliced
- 1 red bell pepper, sliced
- Handful each spinach and kale

Method

1. Mix the chilli powder, smoked paprika, cayenne pepper, and salt in a bowl and evenly sprinkle over the fish fillets.
2. In a large skillet, heat 1 tbsp olive oil until hot. Add the garlic and sauté for 2 minutes.
3. Add the fish fillets to the pan and grill for 5-7 minutes on each side until the fish is cooked. It should easily flake and fall apart with a fork. Set the fish aside.
4. Add the onion and pepper to the pan. Cook for 5 minutes until softened before adding the spinach and kale. Cook for a further 2-3 minutes until the leafy vegetables have wilted.
5. Serve the fish alongside the vegetables and enjoy. If you want to add extra flavour, sprinkle some salt and pepper over the fish or pour some soy sauce onto the vegetables.

Grilled Beef Burger on a Mushroom Bun

Makes 4 servings
Preparation time - 15 minutes
Cooking time - 10 minutes
Nutritional values per serving - 498 kcals, 6 g carbs, 31 g protein, 22 g fat

Ingredients

- 400 g / 14 oz minced beef
- 1 tsp paprika
- 2 tbsp BBQ sauce
- 2 tbsp olive oil
- 4 large mushrooms
- 1 onion, sliced
- 30 g / 1 oz cheddar cheese, grated
- 4 cherry tomatoes, sliced
- Handful lettuce
- 1 avocado, peeled and sliced

Method

1. In a bowl, mix the minced beef, paprika, and BBQ sauce.
2. Form into 4 even patties.
3. Heat 1 tbsp olive oil in a large skillet and cook the mushrooms for 5 minutes on either side until slightly browned and crispy.
4. Remove the mushrooms from the pan and heat the remaining 1 tbsp olive oil in the pan.
5. Add the beef burgers and onion. Cook for 4-5 minutes on either side until the beef has browned and the onions are translucent.
6. Create your burgers by placing the mushrooms on a plate and topping each with a beef burger, some grated cheddar cheese, cherry tomatoes, lettuce, and avocado slices.
7. Add some more BBQ sauce and paprika for extra flavour.

Thai Fish Curry

Makes 4 servings
Preparation time - 10 minutes
Cooking time - 20 minutes
Nutritional values per serving - 256 kcals, 8 g carbs, 19 g protein, 13 g fat

Ingredients

- 1 tbsp coconut oil
- 2 tbsp red curry paste
- 400 ml coconut cream
- 1 tbsp fish sauce
- 400 g white fish fillets, cubed
- 200 g / 7 oz bok choi
- 200 g / 7 oz spinach
- 1 tsp salt

Method

1. Heat 1 tbsp coconut oil in a pan and add the curry paste. Cook for 2-3 minutes on a medium heat.
2. Add the coconut cream and fish sauce to the pan. Bring to a boil before adding the fish and reducing to a simmer for 10 minutes.
3. Add the bok choi and spinach and cook for 3-4 minutes until the vegetables begin to wilt.
4. Serve hot and enjoy.

Chicken Satay

Makes 4 servings
Preparation time - 2 hours 30 minutes
Cooking time - 20 minutes
Nutritional values per serving - 199 kcals, 7 g carbs, 25 g protein, 12 g fat

Ingredients

- 400 g / 14 oz chicken breast fillets, diced
- 3 tbsp smooth peanut butter
- 1 tbsp soy sauce
- 1 tbsp lime juice
- 2 tsp brown sugar
- 2 tbsp chili garlic sauce
- 1 tsp ground ginger

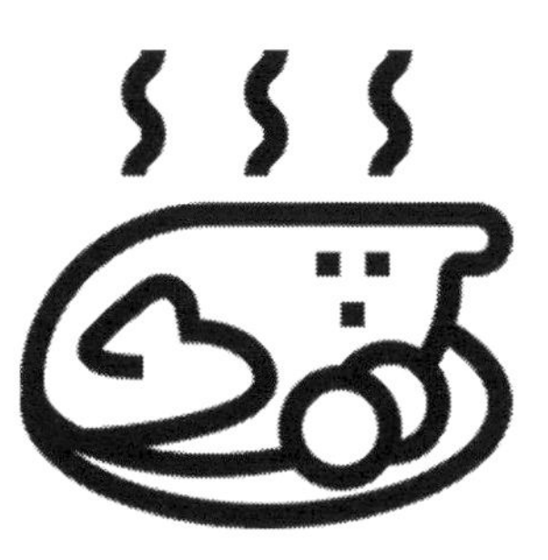

Method

1. Place the diced chicken fillets in a large mixing bowl.
2. In a different bowl, mix all of the remaining ingredients until combined. Pour the peanut satay sauce over the top of the chicken and toss to coat. Cover the bowl with tin foil and set aside to marinate for 2 hours.
3. Drain the chicken, keeping the excess peanut satay sauce.
4. Coat a skillet with cooking oil and place on a high heat. Add the chicken and cook for 12-15 minutes until cooked and golden.
5. Serve immediately with the left-over peanut satay sauce poured over the top. Enjoy with a side of salad and vinaigrette for lunch.

Low-Carb Beef Stew

Makes 4 servings
Preparation time - 15 minutes
Cooking time - 1 hour 30 minutes
Nutritional values per serving - 199 kcals, 7 g carbs, 25 g protein, 12 g fat

Ingredients

- 400 g / 14 oz beef, diced
- 1 tsp salt
- 1 tsp black pepper
- 2 tbsp olive oil
- 400 g / 14 oz mushroom, sliced
- 1 onion, sliced
- 1 carrot, peeled and cut into small pieces
- 2 stalks celery, sliced
- 2 garlic cloves, peeled and minced
- 4 tbsp tomato paste
- 1 tsp dried mixed herbs
- 4 beef stock cubes

Method

1. Season the beef with salt and pepper.
2. Heat the olive oil in a large saucepan and cook the beef in two batches for 4-5 minutes until cooked and golden. Add more oil if necessary.
3. Add the mushrooms and cook for a further 5 minutes. Add the onion, carrot, celery, garlic, tomato paste, and dried mixed herbs. Stir to combine and coat the vegetables.
4. Crumble the stock cubes into the pan and add 600 ml of boiling water. Bring to a boil before reducing the heat and simmering for 60 minutes.
5. Serve the stew piping hot and enjoy!

Meatballs and Zucchini Noodles

Makes 4 servings
Preparation time - 30 minutes
Cooking time - 30 minutes
Nutritional values per serving - 199 kcals, 7 g carbs, 25 g protein, 12 g fat

Ingredients

For the meatballs:

- 450 g / 16 oz turkey, minced
- 1/2 onion, finely sliced
- 1 large egg, beaten
- 100 g / 3.5 oz almond flour
- 1/2 tsp garlic powder
- 1 tbsp sesame seeds

For the glaze:

- 2 tbsp soy sauce
- 1 tsp ground ginger
- 1 tsp honey

For the zucchini noodles:

- 1 tsp olive oil
- 4 zucchinis, spiralised
- 2 garlic cloves, minced
- 1/2 tsp salt

Method

1. To make the meatballs, preheat the oven to 200 °C / 400 °F and line a baking tray with parchment paper.
2. In a large mixing bowl, add the turkey, onion, beaten egg, almond flour, and garlic powder and stir to combine.
3. Roll the mixture into small, evenly sized balls. Place them on the baking tray, keeping them at least 1 inch apart from each other.
4. Bake in the oven for 20 minutes, turning halfway through, until browned.
5. While the meatballs are cooking, make the glaze by mixing all of the ingredients together into a bowl along with the sesame seeds.
6. Heat the sauce for 20-30 seconds in the microwave or for 2-3 minutes in a small pan until warm.
7. Coat the meatballs with the sauce and set aside.
8. To make the zucchini noodles, heat the olive oil in a skillet until hot. Add the spiralised zucchini and garlic and cook until the zucchini begins to release water. Add salt to taste.
9. Divide the zucchini evenly into 4 bowls and top with the meatballs.

Fajita Chicken

Makes 4 servings
Preparation time - 15 minutes
Cooking time - 30 minutes
Nutritional values per serving - 411 kcals, 15 g carbs, 21 g protein, 14 g fat

Ingredients

- 1 tbsp paprika
- 1 tbsp chili powder
- 1 tsp dried chives
- 2 tsp cumin
- 1 tsp salt
- 1 tsp black pepper
- 200 g / 7 oz skinless, boneless chicken breast, sliced
- 1 red pepper, sliced
- 1 yellow pepper, sliced
- 1 onion, sliced
- 2 garlic cloves, peeled and minced
- 2 tbsp olive oil
- 1 tbsp lime juice
- 1 tbsp salsa
- 1 tbsp guacamole

Method

1. Preheat the oven to 180 °C / 350 °F and line a baking tray with parchment paper.
2. Mix the paprika, chili powder, dried chives, cumin, salt, and black pepper in a bowl. Set aside.
3. In a separate bowl, mix the chicken breast, peppers, onion, garlic, olive oil, and lime juice together. Toss to coat the chicken and vegetables in the oil.
4. Spread the chicken and vegetables evenly across the lined baking tray and cook for 25-30 minutes until the chicken is golden and tender, and the vegetables are soft.
5. Remove from the oven and serve with the spices, salsa, and guacamole on top.
6. Low-Carb Desserts and Snacks

Chocolate Mousse

Makes 4 servings
Preparation time - 10 minutes
Cooking time - 10 minutes
Nutritional values per serving - 219 kcals, 10 g carbs, 8 g protein, 19 g fat

Ingredients

- 200 ml whipping cream
- 4 tbsp cocoa powder
- 2 tbsp stevia
- 1 tsp vanilla extract
- 1 tsp cinnamon

Method

1. Whisk the whipping cream into stiff peaks.
2. Fold in the cocoa powder, stevia, vanilla extract, and cinnamon until fully combined.
3. Serve cold as a snack or after dinner.

Low-Carb Cheesecake

Makes 8 servings
Preparation time - 30 minutes
Cooking time - 50 minutes
Nutritional values per serving - 345 kcals, 13 g carbs, 7 g protein, 18 g fat

Ingredients

For the crust:

- 200 g / 7 oz almond flour
- 4 tbsp stevia
- 1 tsp cinnamon
- 6 tbsp butter, melted

For the filling:

- 200 g / 7 oz full fat cream cheese
- 50 g / 1.8 oz sugar
- 4 large eggs, beaten
- 200 g / 7 oz sour cream
- 1 tbsp vanilla extract

Method

1. Preheat the oven to 180 °C / 350 °F and line a round baking tin with parchment paper.
2. To make the crust, mix the almond flour, stevia, and cinnamon in a bowl. Fold in the butter.
3. Pour the mixture into the lined baking tin. Flatten so that the crust is even. Place in the fridge to set for at least 20 minutes.
4. Meanwhile, mix the filling ingredients in a bowl until fully combined.
5. Remove the crust from the fridge and pour the filling on top. Spread the filling so that it is even and flat on top.
6. Serve the cheesecake with a side of whipped cream.

Unsweetened Homemade Trail Mix

Makes 4 servings
Preparation time - 5 minutes
Cooking time - none
Nutritional values per serving - 212 kcals, 7 g carbs, 16 g protein, 30 g fat

Ingredients

- 50 g / 1.8 oz pumpkin seeds
- 50 g / 1.8 oz sunflower seeds
- 100 g / 3.5 oz pecans, chopped
- 100 g / 3.5 oz walnuts, chopped
- 30 g / 1 oz coconut flakes

Method

1. Preheat the oven to 180 °C / 350 °F and line a baking tray with parchment paper.
2. Spread the pumpkin seeds and sunflower seeds evenly across the tray.
3. Roast the seeds for 10-15 minutes until crunchy and golden.
4. Place the seeds in a bowl and mix in the nuts and coconut flakes.
5. Enjoy!

Dark Chocolate and Almond Bark

Makes 8 servings
Preparation time - 20 minutes
Cooking time - 10 minutes
Nutritional values per serving - 156 kcals, 12 g carbs, 16 g protein, 17 g fat

Ingredients

- 200 g / 7 oz dark chocolate (at least 75% cocoa)
- 100 g / 3.5 oz almonds
- 50 g / 1.8 oz pumpkin seeds
- 50 g / 1.8 oz sunflower seeds

Method

1. Line a baking tray with parchment paper.
2. Chop the chocolate into small pieces and place into a heat proof bowl. Place the bowl on top of a small saucepan filled with water.
3. Heat the saucepan to a simmer and allow the chocolate to melt, stirring occasionally.
4. When half of the chocolate has fully melted, remove the bowl from the heat and set aside.
5. When the chocolate has cooled down slightly but is still warm, stir in the almonds, pumpkin seeds, and sunflower seeds.
6. Spread the chocolate across the lined tray and smooth the top so that it is even. Place in the fridge for 10-15 minutes to harden.
7. Once hardened, cut the bark into 8 servings, and enjoy.

Kale Chips

Makes 4 servings
Preparation time - 5 minutes
Cooking time - 15 minutes
Nutritional values per serving - 87 kcals, 5 g carbs, 3 g protein, 5 g fat

Ingredients

- 200 g / 7 oz kale
- 1 tbsp coconut oil
- 1 tsp chili powder
- 1 tsp cumin

Method

1. Preheat the oven to 200 °C / 400 °F and line a baking tray with parchment paper.
2. Rinse the kale and allow to dry. Tear into small pieces and discard the stems.
3. Place the kale in a mixing bowl and toss in the coconut oil and spices to coat.
4. Spread the kale evenly over the baking tray and bake in the oven for 15 minutes until crispy and brown.
5. Serve immediately and store any leftovers in an airtight container.

Low-Carb Choc Chip Cookies

Makes 8 servings
Preparation time - 15 minutes
Cooking time - 15 minutes
Nutritional values per serving - 213 kcals, 8 g carbs, 5 g protein, 10 g fat

Ingredients

- 2 large eggs, beaten
- 50 g / 1.8 oz butter
- 2 tbsp heavy cream
- 1 tsp vanilla extract
- 1 tsp cinnamon
- 200 g / 7 oz almond flour
- 2 tbsp stevia
- 50 g / 1.8 oz dark chocolate, broken into small pieces

Method

1. Preheat the oven to 200 °C / 400 °F and line a baking tray with parchment paper.
2. In a bowl, mix the eggs, butter, heavy cream, vanilla extract, and cinnamon until fully combined.
3. Fold in the almond flour, stevia, and chocolate chips.
4. Roll the mixture into small, even balls and flatten into cookies on the lined baking tray.
5. Bake in the oven for 15 minutes until golden and crispy.

Low-Carb Chocolate Mug Cake

Makes 1 serving
Preparation time - 5 minutes
Cooking time - 5 minutes
Nutritional values per serving - 398 kcals, 10 g carbs, 10 g protein, 14 g fat

Ingredients

- 2 tbsp butter, melted
- 100 g / 3.5 oz almond flour
- 1 tbsp cocoa powder
- 50 g / 1.8 oz dark chocolate chips
- 1 large egg, beaten
- ½ tsp baking powder
- 50 ml whipped cream

Method

1. Mix all of the ingredients in a bowl, except the whipped cream.
2. Pour the mixture into a microwave-safe mug and heat in the microwave for 45-60 seconds until the cake is set, but still soft.
3. Serve while warm with some whipped cream on top.

Low-Carb Chocolate and Peanut Butter Cookies

Makes 8 servings
Preparation time - 5 minutes
Cooking time - none
Nutritional values per serving - 212 kcals, 12 g carbs, 12 g protein, 16 g fat

Ingredients

- 100 g / 3.5 oz smooth peanut butter
- 100 g / 3.5 oz crunchy peanut butter
- 200 g / 7 oz coconut flour
- 3 tbsp stevia
- 1 tsp vanilla extract
- 50 g / 1.8 oz dark chocolate chips
- 2 tbsp coconut oil

Method

1. Line a baking tray with parchment paper.
2. In a bowl, mix both the smooth and crunchy peanut butter, coconut flour, stevia, and vanilla until all of the ingredients are fully combined.
3. Use a tablespoon to scoop small parts of the mixture and roll them into small balls. Try to keep each ball a similar size.
4. Place the balls on the lined baking tray and flatten slightly.
5. In a small microwave-safe bowl, mix the chocolate chips and coconut oil until combined. Place in the microwave for 30-60 seconds, stopping to stir every 10 seconds, until the chocolate has fully melted.
6. Pour the hot chocolate and coconut oil mixture over the peanut butter balls until fully coated.
7. Drizzle a little more peanut butter over the top of the balls if desired and store in the freezer for at least 1 hour to set.
8. Serve cold and store any leftovers in the freezer.

Chocolate Protein Shake

Makes 1 serving
Preparation time - 5 minutes
Cooking time - none
Nutritional values per serving - 250 kcals, 8 g carbs, 26 g protein, 16 g fat

Ingredients

- 200 ml almond milk
- 1 scoop chocolate protein powder
- 2 tbsp almond butter
- 1 tbsp cocoa powder
- 2 tsp stevia
- 2 tbsp chia seeds
- 1 tsp vanilla extract

Method

1. Place all of the ingredients into a blender or food processor.
2. Blend until a smooth and consistent mixture has formed.
3. Pour the protein shake into a cup and enjoy!

Cinnamon Mug Cake

Makes 1 serving
Preparation time - 5 minutes
Cooking time - none
Nutritional values per serving - 142 kcals, 7 g carbs, 12 g protein, 12 g fat

Ingredients

- 4 tbsp almond flour
- 2 tsp cinnamon
- 1/2 tsp baking powder
- 1 tbsp sugar
- 1 egg, beaten
- 100 ml oat milk

Method

1. Grease a large microwave-safe mug with butter.
2. Mix all of the ingredients in a bowl until fully combined. Pour into the greased mug.
3. Cook in the microwave for 45-60 seconds until the cake is set but still slightly soft.
4. Serve while the mug cake is still warm with an extra sprinkle of cinnamon and a side of whipped cream.

14 Days Low-Carb Meal Plan

Day 1

Breakfast - Sausage Sandwich

Makes 2 servings

Preparation time - 10 minutes

Cooking time - 20 minutes

Nutritional values per serving - 236 kcals, 12 g carbs, 20 g protein, 16 g fat

Ingredients

- 4 large eggs
- 2 tbsp heavy cream
- 1/2 tsp salt
- 1/2 tsp black pepper
- 1 tbsp butter
- 30 g / 1 oz cheddar cheese, sliced
- 4 sausage patties
- 1 avocado

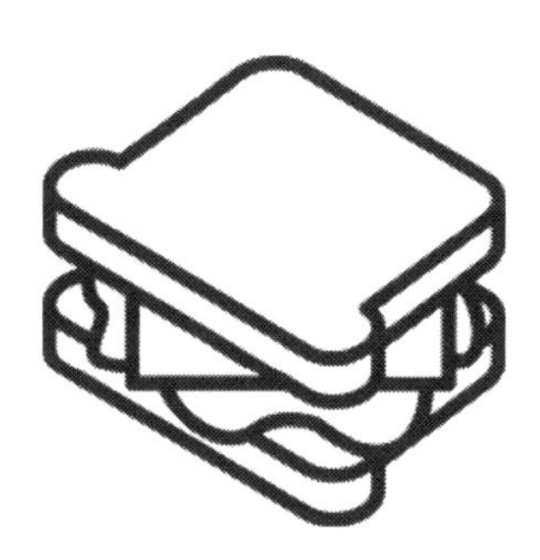

Method

1. Preheat the oven to 200 °C / 400 °F and line a baking tray with parchment paper. Cook the sausage patties for 20 minutes until cooked, turning half way through.
2. Meanwhile, crack the eggs into a bowl and add the heavy cream, salt, and pepper. Whisk until fully combined
3. Heat a skillet and add the butter to melt. Pour half of the egg mixture into the hot skillet and add ½ of the cheese slices into the centre of the egg mixture.
4. Allow the eggs and cheese to cook for 1-2 minutes before folding the sides of the eggs over the cheese.
5. Repeat with the other half of the eggs and cheese.
6. Remove the sausage patties from the oven and place them on a plate. Add an egg each onto 2 of the patties, and top with the remaining two patties to form a sandwich.

Lunch - Deliciously Devilled Eggs (See page 35)

Dinner - Steak and Cheese Stuffed Peppers (See page 52)

Day 2

Breakfast - Keto Bagels ***(See page 26)***

Lunch - Low-Carb Egg Salad

Makes 4 servings

Preparation time - 15 minutes

Cooking time - 20 minutes

Nutritional values per serving - 165 kcals, 10 g carbs, 15 g protein, 12 g fat

Ingredients

- 6 large eggs
- 1 tsp olive oil
- 2 slices bacon
- 3 tbsp mayonnaise
- 1 tsp lemon juice
- 1 tbsp dried herbs
- 1/2 tsp black pepper
- 1 avocado
- Handful lettuce
- 4 cherry tomatoes, halved

Method

1. Heat a saucepan of water and bring to boil. Reduce the heat to a light simmer and add the eggs. Turn the heat back up to boil and cook the eggs for 10-12 minutes.
2. Meanwhile, heat 1 tsp olive oil in a skillet and add the bacon slices. Cook for 10 minutes, turning halfway through until the bacon turns slightly brown and crispy. Once cooked, set aside to drain on paper towels.
3. Remove the eggs from the pan once cooked and set aside to cool.
4. When the eggs are cooled, peel the skins, chop into small pieces, and place in a bowl.
5. Chop the bacon into small slices and add to the eggs along with the mayonnaise, lemon juice, dried herbs, and black pepper.
6. Peel the skin off the avocado and slice in half. Remove the pit and chop the two avocado halves into small chunks.
7. Add the avocado to the bowl and mix until the ingredients are fully combined.
8. Serve the low-carb egg salad evenly onto 4 plates alongside a handful of lettuce and the cherry tomato halves.

Dinner - Spicy Fish Taco Bowls (See page 56)

Day 3

Breakfast - Low-Carb Breakfast Waffles ***(See page 22)***

Lunch - Chicken and Veggie Bowls ***(See page 34)***

Dinner - Soy and Honey Salmon

Makes 4 servings

Preparation time - 20 minutes

Cooking time - 10 minutes

Nutritional values per serving - 301 kcals, 6 g carbs, 20 g protein, 19 g fat

Ingredients

- 400 g / 14 oz salmon fillets
- 2 tbsp soy sauce
- 1 tbsp honey
- 1 onion, finely sliced

Method

1. Preheat the oven to 200 °C / 400 °F and line a baking tray with parchment paper.
2. In a bowl, mix the soy sauce, honey, and sliced onion in a bowl until combined.
3. Carefully place the salmon fillets on the baking tray and pour the sauce evenly over the top of each fillet.
4. and cook in the oven for 15-20 minutes until the fish flakes easily when pressed with a fork.
5. Serve with a side of roasted low-carb vegetables and enjoy!

Day 4

Breakfast - Keto Pancakes

Makes 4 servings

Preparation time - 5 minutes

Cooking time - 10 minutes

Nutritional values per serving - 404 kcals, 8 g carbs, 14 g protein, 23 g fat

Ingredients

- 2 large eggs, beaten
- 50 g / 2 oz cream cheese
- 100 g / 3.5 oz almond flour
- 1 tsp baking powder
- 2 tsp vanilla extract
- 2 tsp dried cinnamon

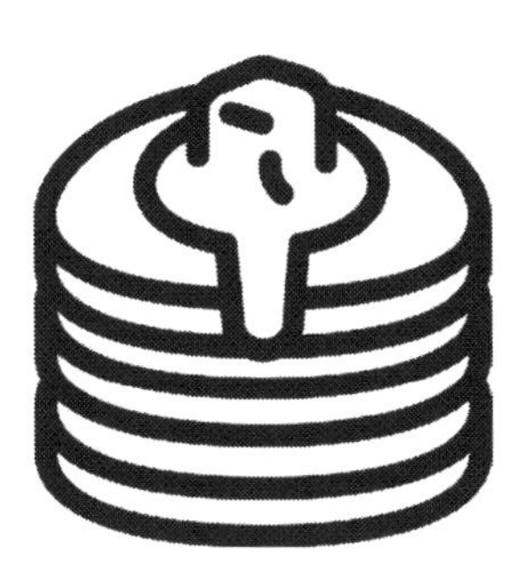

Method

1. Place all of the ingredients in a bowl and whisk until fully combined.
2. Let the batter sit for a couple of minutes while you heat a frying pan over a medium heat.
3. Pour one-quarter of the batter into the hot pan and allow to spread into a pancake.
4. Cook the pancake until you begin to see bubbles forming in the batter and flip onto the other side. Continue cooking for a further 2-3 minutes until both sides are cooked.
5. Repeat a further 3 times with the rest of the pancake batter
6. Serve with some butter and a small dash of syrup. Be careful not to use too much syrup as it contains a lot of sugars.

Lunch - Stuffed Avocados (See page 44)

Dinner - Meatballs and Zucchini Noodles (See page 65)

Day 5

Breakfast - Bacon and Egg Rolls ***(See page 24)***

Lunch - Low-Fat Hash

Makes 4 servings

Preparation time - 15 minutes

Cooking time - 25 minutes

Nutritional values per serving - 181 kcals, 5 g carbs, 11 g protein, 9 g fat

Ingredients

- 2 tbsp olive oil
- 1 turnip, peeled and diced
- 100 g / 3.5 oz brussel sprouts, halved
- 100 g / 3.5 oz asparagus, cut into pieces
- 1 onion, sliced
- 1 tsp garlic powder
- 1 tsp paprika
- 1/2 salt
- 1/2 black pepper
- 4 large eggs

Method

1. Heat the olive oil in a skillet over medium heat.
2. Add the turnip, brussel sprouts, asparagus, and onion. Cook until the vegetables begin to soften and become fragrant.
3. Add the garlic powder, paprika, salt, and pepper and continue cooking for a further 30 seconds.
4. Create 4 holes in the hash mixture and crack an egg into each. Cook for 10 minutes until the egg whites are fully cooked.

Dinner - Chicken Satay (See page 61)

Day 6

Breakfast - Vegetable Frittata ***(See page 28)***

Lunch - Tuscan Salmon ***(See page 48)***

Dinner - Peanut Butter Chicken

Makes 4 servings

Preparation time - 10 minutes

Cooking time - 30 minutes

Nutritional values per serving - 467 kcals, 7 g carbs, 21 g protein, 23 g fat

Ingredients

- 2 tbsp olive oil
- 8 skinless, boneless chicken thighs, cut into chunks
- 1 onion, finely chopped
- 3 garlic cloves, crushed
- 2 tsp dried garlic
- 2 tsp dried ginger
- 2 tbsp garam masala
- 100 g / 3.5 oz peanut butter, smooth or crunchy
- 400 ml coconut milk
- 400 g / 14 oz canned tomatoes
- 1 tsp coriander

Method

1. Heat 1 olive oil in a large frying pan over medium heat.
2. Add the chicken thigh chunks and cook for 15-20 minutes until the chicken begins to turn golden brown. Remove the chicken from the pan and set aside to drain on paper towels.
3. Add the onions and garlic cloves and cook for 5 minutes.
4. Add the dried garlic, dried ginger, and garam masala, along with the remaining tbsp olive oil.
5. Cook for 1 further minute before adding the peanut butter, coconut milk, and chopped tomatoes. Stir to coat the chicken and bring to simmer.
6. Return the chicken thighs to the pan and sprinkle in the coriander. Heat for a few more minutes until all of the ingredients are hot.
7. Serve up the peanut butter chicken with some steamed vegetables.

Day 7

Breakfast - Keto Pork Breakfast Cups

Makes 3 servings

Preparation time - 15 minutes

Cooking time - 20 minutes

Nutritional values per serving - 315 kcals, 9 g carbs, 16 g protein, 12 g fat

Ingredients

- 400 g / 14 oz ground pork
- 1 tbsp dried thyme
- 2 cloves garlic, minced
- 1 tsp paprika
- 1 tsp salt
- ½ tsp black pepper
- 50 g / 1.8 oz fresh spinach
- 50 g / 1.8 oz cheddar cheese, grated
- 4 eggs

Method

1. Preheat the oven to 200 °C / 400 °F and line a 6-piece muffin tray with cases.
2. In a mixing bowl, combine the ground pork, thyme, garlic cloves, paprika, salt, and black pepper until fully combined.
3. Place a small amount of minced pork into each baking case and press down to create a base. Spread the spinach evenly across all six muffin cases and then crack one egg into each.
4. Bake in the oven for 20 to 25 minutes until the eggs are cooked and the muffins are warm.
5. To serve, place 2 cups on your plate alongside a handful of salad or low-carb vegetables.

Lunch - Steak Bites and Zucchini Noodles (See page 37)

Dinner - Grilled Beef Burger on a Mushroom Bun (See page 58)

Day 8

Breakfast - Strawberry and Avocado Low-Fat Smoothie ***(See page 30)***

Lunch - Hot and Spicy Shrimp Lettuce Wraps

Makes 4 servings
Preparation time - 15 minutes
Cooking time - 5 minutes
Nutritional values per serving - 225 kcals, 4 g carbs, 12 g protein, 8 g fat

Ingredients

- 400 g / 14 oz shrimp, peeled, deveined, and tails removed
- 1 tbsp hot sauce
- 1 tbsp olive oil
- 1 head lettuce, separated into large leaves
- 1/2 red onion, finely sliced
- 4 cherry tomatoes, halved
- 50 g / 1.8 oz cheddar cheese, grated

Method

1. Place the shrimp in a bowl and toss in the hot sauce.
2. Heat 1 tbsp olive in a pan and add the shrimp. Cook for 2-3 minutes on each side.
3. Assemble the wraps by placing the large lettuce leaves on a plate. Evenly spread the cooked shrimp between the leaves before topping with chopped onion, halved cherry tomatoes, and grated cheddar cheese.
4. Add a dash of extra hot sauce if desired and enjoy!

Dinner - Steak and Cheese Stuffed Peppers ***(See page 52)***

Day 9

Breakfast - Cashew Butter Breakfast Pots ***(See page 31)***

Lunch - Stuffed Avocados ***(See page 44)***

Dinner - Creamy Garlic Salmon

Makes 4 servings

Preparation time - 10 minutes

Cooking time - 15 minutes

Nutritional values per serving - 346 kcals, 10 g carbs, 17 g protein, 13 g fat

Ingredients

- 2 tbsp olive oil
- 400 g salmon fillets
- 200 g / 7 oz heavy cream
- 1 tsp garlic powder
- 1 tsp dried mixed herbs
- Zest 1 lemon
- 50 g / 1.8 oz Parmesan cheese, grated
- 100 g / 3.5 oz fresh spinach, chopped

Method

1. Heat 2 tbsp olive in a frying pan and add the salmon fillets. Cook for 3-5 minutes on each side until browned.
2. Once cooked, set aside. Place in a pre-heated oven to keep warm. Alternatively, keep the salmon warm on a very low heat in the pan.
3. Make the sauce by combining the heavy cream, garlic powder, mixed herbs, and zest of 1 lemon in a saucepan.
4. Heat over a low heat, stirring frequently. Add the spinach and continue to heat until the spinach wilts.
5. Serve the salmon warm with the creamy garlic sauce poured over the top. Add a side of low-carb vegetables.

Day 10

Breakfast - Low-Carb Avocado Toast

Makes 1 serving
Preparation time - 10 time
Cooking - 2 minutes
Nutritional values per serving - 289 kcals, 10 g carbs, 7 g protein, 12 g fat

Ingredients

- 1 avocado
- 2 slices keto bread
- Juice 1 lemon
- 1/2 tsp black pepper

Method

1. Remove the skin and the pit from the avocado and slice.
2. Place the keto bread in the toaster and cook to your desired crispness.
3. When the toast is ready, add the avocado slices and squirt the lemon juice on top. Add a sprinkle of black pepper and serve while the bread is still hot.

Lunch - Chicken and Veggie Bowls (See page 34)

Dinner - Low-Carb Beef Stew (See page 63)

Day 11

Breakfast - Vegetable Frittata ***(See page 28)***

Lunch - Cauliflower Mac and Cheese

Makes 2 servings

Preparation time - 15 minutes

Cooking time - 30 minutes

Nutritional values per serving - 345 kcals, 12 kcals, 6 g protein, 17 g fat

Ingredients

- 1 large cauliflower, broken into florets
- 1 tbsp butter
- 1 onion, sliced
- 3 tbsp almond flour
- 200 ml milk
- 100 g / 3.5 oz cheddar cheese, grated
- 1 tsp black pepper

Method

1. Preheat the oven to 200 °C / 400 °F and line a small casserole dish with parchment paper. Bring a large saucepan of water to boil and add the cauliflower. Cook for 7-8 minutes until softened. Drain and set aside.
2. Heat 1 tbsp butter in a frying pan and add the onion. Cook for 5 minutes until they start to become fragrant and brown.
3. Stir the flour into the pan and reduce the heat. Continue cooking for 3-4 minutes until the flour is absorbed.
4. Add the milk to the pan and bring to boil. Simmer until the milk thickens.
5. Once the milk has thickened, remove from the heat, and stir in the cheddar cheese.
6. Stir the cauliflower into the pan and mix to coat in the sauce.
7. Pour into the lined casserole dish and bake in the oven for 20 minutes until the Mac and cheese is hot all the way through and crispy on top.
8. Serve hot with a side salad.

Dinner - Soy and Honey Salmon (See page 87)

Day 12

Breakfast - Strawberry and Avocado Low-Fat Smoothie (See page 30)

Lunch - Bacon Sushi Rolls (See page 43)

Dinner - Garlic Chicken Meatballs and Cauliflower Rice

Makes 4 servings

Preparation time - 15 minutes

Cooking time - 15 minutes

Nutritional values per serving - 321 kcals, 11 g carbs, 18 g protein, 14 g fat

Ingredients

- 1 cauliflower, broken into florets
- 400 g / 14 oz skinless, boneless chicken, ground
- 100 g / 7 oz cheddar cheese, grated
- 4 cloves garlic, peeled and minced
- 1 tsp Italian herbs
- 2 chicken stock cubes, dissolved
- 2 tbsp olive oil
- Juice 1 lemon
- 1 tbsp hot sauce

Method

1. Make the cauliflower rice by adding the florets to a blender or food processor. Pulse until the cauliflower is completely broken down and resembles rice.
2. Transfer the cauliflower to a bowl, add around 200 ml water, and cook in the microwave for 4-5 minutes until all of the water has been absorbed.
3. In a large bowl, mix the ground chicken, cheese, garlic, and Italian herbs until the chicken is well coated.
4. Scoop small chunks of the chicken mixture to form meatballs.
5. Heat 2 tbsp olive oil in a large frying pan and cook the meatballs for 10 minutes until brown and crispy, turning over halfway through. Remove from the pan and set aside on paper towels.
6. Add the lemon juice and hot sauce to the bowl containing the cauliflower rice and mix well.
7. Serve the meatballs on a bed of cauliflower rice and enjoy.

Day 13

Breakfast - No Oats Oatmeal

Makes 1 serving

Preparation time - 5 minutes

Cooking time - 5 minutes

Nutritional values per serving - 198 kcals, 5 g carbs, 7 g protein, 8 g fat

Ingredients

- 1 tbsp almond flour
- 1 tbsp desiccated coconut
- 2 tbsp flaxseed
- 1 tbsp chia seeds
- 1/2 tsp stevia
- 1/2 tsp vanilla extract
- Handful blueberries
- 1/2 tsp cinnamon

Method

1. Combine all of the ingredients in a bowl.
2. Transfers the mixture into a saucepan. Cook the oatmeal over a low heat for 4-5 minutes until thickened.
3. Serve while hot with some fresh blueberries and a sprinkle of cinnamon

Lunch - Avocado, Egg, and Tomato Salad (See page 39)

Dinner - Fajita Chicken (See page 67)

Day 14

Breakfast - Keto Pork Breakfast Cups ***(See page 94)***

Lunch - Cauliflower Potato Salad

Makes 4 servings

Preparation time - 5 minutes

Cooking time - 10 minutes

Nutritional values per serving - 257 kcals, 8 g carbs, 6 g protein, 12 g fat

Ingredients

- 1 large cauliflower, broken into florets
- 2 eggs
- 1 tbsp mayonnaise
- 1 tbsp olive oil
- 1 tsp Dijon mustard
- 1 tsp white vinegar
- 1 tsp cumin
- 1 tsp smoked paprika
- 1/2 tsp salt
- 1/2 tsp black pepper
- 1/2 red onion, sliced

Method

1. Bring a saucepan of water to boil and add the cauliflower. Cook for 8-10 minutes until softened. Drain and set aside to cool slightly.
2. Meanwhile, heat a second pan of water to a simmer and add the eggs. Cook for 10 minutes to create hardboiled eggs. Set aside to cool before peeling the eggs and slicing them in half.
3. In a bowl combine, the remaining ingredients. Add the cauliflower to the bowl and toss to fully coat.
4. Evenly spread the cauliflower between 4 bowls and add half a hard-boiled egg to each.

Dinner - Spicy Fish Taco Bowls (See page 107)

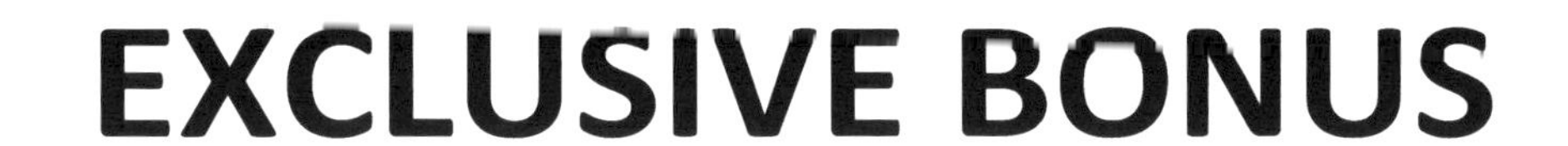

EXCLUSIVE BONUS

40 Weight Loss Recipes

&

14 Days Meal Plan

Scan the QR-Code and receive
the FREE download:

Disclaimer

This book contains opinions and ideas of the author and is meant to teach the reader informative and helpful knowledge while due care should be taken by the user in the application of the information provided. The instructions and strategies are possibly not right for every reader and there is no guarantee that they work for everyone. Using this book and implementing the information/recipes therein contained is explicitly your own responsibility and risk. This work with all its contents, does not guarantee correctness, completion, quality or correctness of the provided information. Misinformation or misprints cannot be completely eliminated.

Printed in Great Britain
by Amazon